# How to Lose Weight Without Really Dieting

I0422898

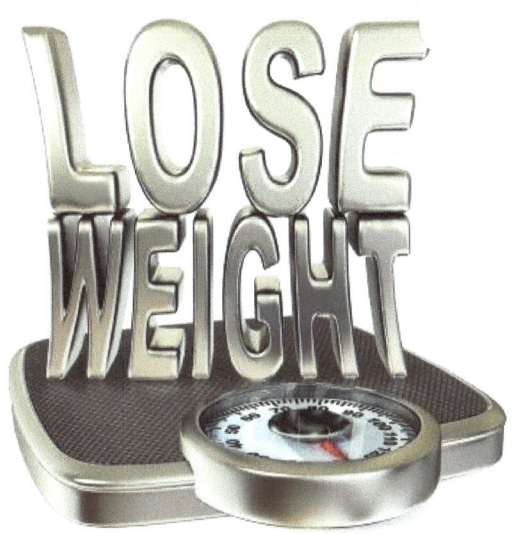

**Dueep J Singh**

**Health Learning Series**

**Mendon Cottage Books**

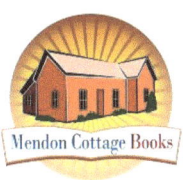

*JD-Biz Publishing*

**Download Free Books!**

http://MendonCottageBooks.com

## Disclaimer

The information is this book is provided for informational purposes only. It is not intended to be used and medical advice or a substitute for proper medical treatment by a qualified health care provider. The information is believed to be accurate as presented based on research by the author.

The contents have not been evaluated by the U.S. Food and Drug Administration or any other Government or Health Organization and the contents in this book are not to be used to treat cure or prevent disease.

The author or publisher is not responsible for the use or safety of any diet, procedure or treatment mentioned in this book. The author or publisher is not responsible for errors or omissions that may exist.

## Warning

The Book is for informational purposes only and before taking on any diet, treatment or medical procedure it is recommended to consult with your primary care provider.

Our books are available at

1. Amazon.com

2. Barnes and Noble

3. Itunes

4. Kobo

5. Smashwords

6. Google Play Books

# Table of Contents

Introduction ............................................................................... 4

How does Dieting Harm Your Body? .......................................... 9

How Do Eating Habits Inculcated In Childhood Affect Us As Long As We Live? ......................................................................................... 12

Why Do You Need To Lose Weight? ........................................ 14

SO NOW WE COME TO HOW TO LOSE WEIGHT WITHOUT REALLY DIETING ...................................................................... 16

    Re-educate your eating habits ................................................. 18

    The second principle is – losing weight is done slowly and has to be done slowly ................................................................................ 18

Easy Tips and Techniques to Remain Slim and Trim ................. 27

    Let us help you get started with easy tips and techniques to remain Slim and trim. ............................................................................ 27

Conclusion ............................................................................. 32

Author Bio .............................................................................. 33

Publisher ................................................................................ 44

# Introduction

Have you noticed that at a get-together or a party, when the conversation starts to lag, there is one health-conscious person who starts the conversational ball rolling again with just one sentence "I have found a really amazing diet, which helps me to lose weight really fast." And then you can see the sound volume increase, as everybody within hearing distance is going to start clamoring about their own weight problem, how they are looking for the best diets to lose weight, how they have been trying to implement the strict regime, and whether they are getting to be successful in their endeavors or not…

And then we look at the food…

**And the end result is –**

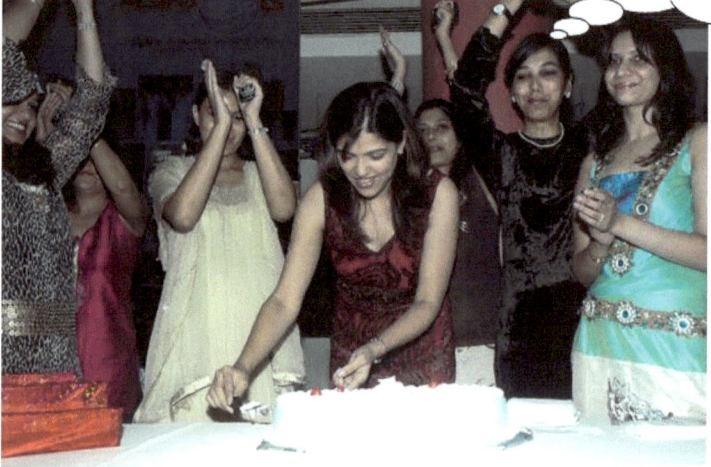

*Well that may be you smiling bravely but your diet regime went out of the window the moment you saw that cake. I know that I cannot resist all the tempting goodies at a party. And neither can you. In fact, neither SHOULD YOU! If your health allows you to eat and drink what you want, indulge yourself while you can!*

*So this book is about, How we can enjoy the good things in life (Food, glorious food, and drink and yet not feel guilty about enjoying them) and still lose weight...*

This is what we have found out when a person goes on a strict diet to lose weight.

- We are never happy with the end results ever.

- Many of these weight loss programs may give us a temporary satisfying result, but we find ourselves in gaining weight after a while.

- Many of these fads which promise us immediate weight loss have a detrimental long-term effect on our bodies.

- It is very difficult for us to restrict ourselves to just one weight loss program, when there is another weight loss program recommended by our favorite movie stars or talk-show hosts… And so on.

You and I come in this category, because we have our own weight loss and weight gain stories and trials to tell. That is because this new generation is so weight conscious, that we try our best to get rid of that extra weight, almost overnight, when it took about 3 to 4 years for us to abuse our body so much that it started to gain that weight.

So, before I tell you how to lose weight without really dieting, let us go back to the reasons why people of the 20th and 21st century are so obsessed with weight.

Look at the paintings done by Rubens. All his models are chubby and in 20th century terms, the females are distinctly obese and so are the babies.

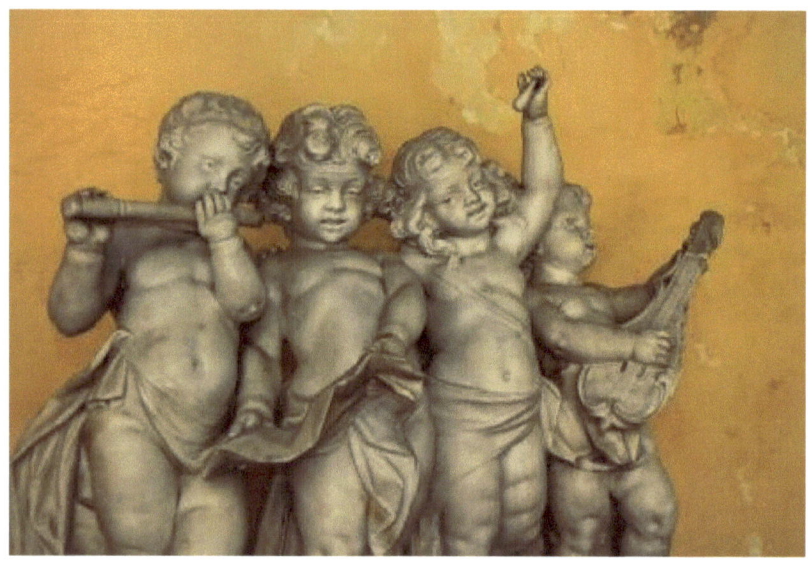

**Even the cherubs are fat...**

That is because at that time, the idea of being fat was considered to be the epitome of beauty brought on by having enough to eat. In the same way, the aristocrats were always fat unless they were warriors with their bodies well-honed to keep them fighting fit. Only very prosperous people with plenty to eat could afford to be fat. The rest of the majority was lean and thin, because it was the time of survival of the fittest. If you did not work hard, you did not eat for the day. And this continuous physical exercise kept people lean and thin.

*Eat drink and be merry 'cause we know not how to diet.*

On the other hand, as soon as the standard of living started to improve from the 19th century onwards, due to better farming knowledge and tools, people stopped worrying about having enough food, because there was plentiful fare which was easily available. Hard physical exercise also started taking a backseat because changing lifestyle ensured that people did not have to work so hard physically. So they began to put on weight, because all they had to do is relax, sit and eat.

Eating without exercise gave rise to many health problems. It is only in the 20th century that people began to know that many of these health problems were related to their diets, and to that extra weight.

That extra layer of fat which we want removed from the body is genetically provided to us by nature, so that we can keep warm. There was a time when our ancestors blessed that insulating layer of blubber, because it prevented the internal organs from being damaged in cold weather. Their 2000 times descendants curse it because they think that retracts from their own modern idea of beauty and attractiveness. That is because the modern epitome of beauty, handsomeness and fitness is a slim, trim body without an ounce of fat on it.

How many times have you read some book, when the heroine's eyes bug out when she catches sight of the hero's lean, mean fighting machine silhouette, quote, without an ounce of fat on it, unquote. That is because he is used to working hard physically or working out regularly. He is the hero, but in real life?

We are normal basically lazy human beings. We just hate exerting ourselves physically.

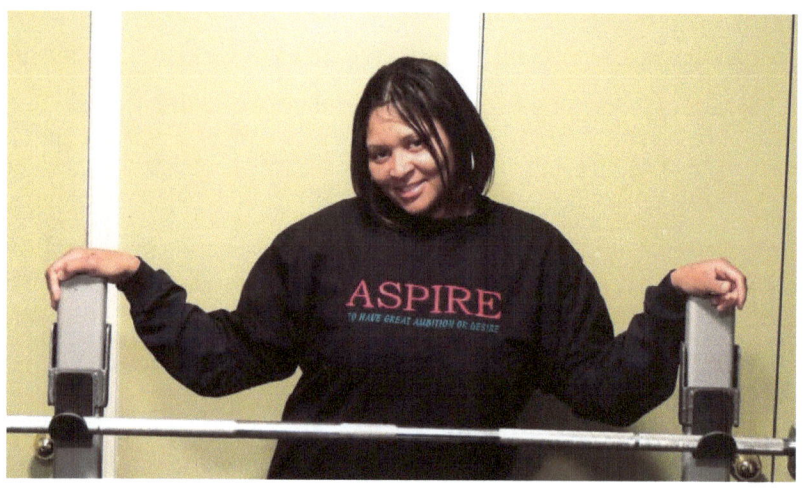

*We hate the idea of exercise. We hate the idea of dieting. All that hassle is such a bore. Natasha may love exercising but I don't and I am sure you don't either! (Photo courtesy: Natasha Chase)*

This book is to give you amazing tips and techniques on how to lose weight without dieting, how to keep healthy throughout your life with sensible lifestyle tips, and how to use this knowledge to keep healthy, fit and fine as long as you live.

# How does Dieting Harm Your Body?

Whenever I see a perfectly healthy person moaning about she or he needs to lose weight, I know what is going to come next. They want to talk about their latest diet, they want to talk about how gaining weight has lessened their self-esteem, or they are comparing themselves with some stick insects who they consider to be attractive and they want to be exactly like those unhealthy specimens.

I want to shake them and tell them, "Why do you need to lose weight? You are perfectly healthy, at the moment, according to what I can see. However, if you change your body physiology and natural chemical makeup by creating an artificial imbalance, through embarking on a diet, you are going to lose out in the long run. "

But many of us are stubborn. We have to prove to ourselves that if something worked for Victoria Beckham or Naomi Campbell, it is going to work for us. Victoria is definitely not healthy. She has nearly starved herself to dangerous, potentially life-threatening levels. Naomi Campbell's occasional outbursts of bad temper should give everybody a signal "she has embarked upon another diet to lose weight. This has a detrimental effect on her mind, body as well as on her temper, because the body is not getting essential nutrients needed to keep working properly as nature intended it to do.

That is why it is sending out "I need food, I need healthy, nourishing health restoring food right now." And she is ignoring that message because according to her, her public appeal is related to her pencil thin silhouette. So she is going to starve her rather than having some critic say "Naomi has gained a bit of weight." This statement in itself is conducive enough for her to start drastic dieting right now. This leads to bad tempered displays in public and possible aggressive behavior in the future, as long as she keeps starving herself.

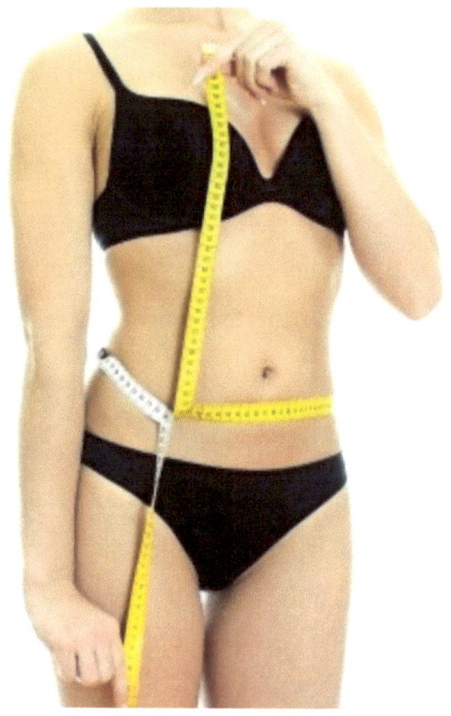

**If you find yourself doing this exercise with a tape measure every day-Stop. Cease. Desist. This is conducive to tension, obsessing about weight loss, and weight gain. This may also lead to bad eating habits and bulimia/anorexia.**

Do not ever let you encourage that sort of mindset ever. Once you start thinking about what the public expects from you, instead of thinking of your own body, you have had it. Your state of good natural health should not be compromised ever, because your body is used to a set of natural health giving nutrients in order to keep healthy. The moment you start depriving it of these nutrients, the buyer physiological makeup starts to change in order to compensate for this deprivation. This leads to a slow and steady deprivation.

# How Do Eating Habits Inculcated In Childhood Affect Us As Long As We Live?

Sedentary lifestyles and eating unhealthy food over a given period of time have left a number of us distinctly unhealthy. Just look around you. How many children do you see are really healthy in your neighborhood? How many of these children are touching the border line of obesity? Do you know that 49% of American children have become vulnerable to possible bad health risks in the future, because of their bad eating habits?

On the other hand, a large number of children all over the world are suffering from malnutrition, because they do not have access to healthy diets. That means they are going to suffer throughout their lives from disease brought about by malnutrition.

In the 30s, 40s, and 50s, mothers were very careful about proper diet. Children were encouraged to go out and play baseball, football, and do other physical activities. Then they came back home as healthy as young bears to be given well-balanced, healthy, and nourishing food, which consisted of proteins, carbohydrates, fats, minerals, and other essential nutrients. That was if their mothers knew about healthy diets. These children are still comparatively healthy, even though they are in their 60s, 70s and 80s now. That is because they were not exposed to potential health risks starting from childhood itself. However, children today are encouraged to sit in front of a TV or to play computer games indoors in order to keep them quiet. Very few mothers tell them to get out and breathe some fresh air. Many Mothers would rather encourage children to eat whatever is in the fridge, than prepare something which is healthy.

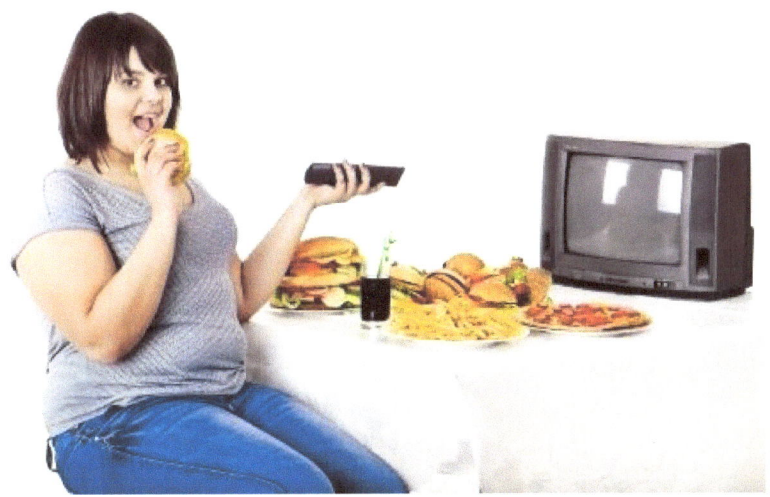

**The age of Fast food and TV Dinners...**

End result- unhealthy, obese kids

In the East, the traditional idea of showing how much you care for your family is to cook lots of good food for them and encourage them to eat and eat and eat. That is why a number of children who are stuffed like turkeys in childhood grow distinctly plump before they are 10. And the mothers are satisfied because the neighbors call them good mothers taking good care of their families. Each one from father to baby is definitely spherical in shape. What they are not going to tell the mother is that not only is she harming her family, but she is leaving them prone to future ill health.

# Why Do You Need To Lose Weight?

Remember the days when you were thin? You seemed to be bubbling with energy. You bustled energetically from place to place without feeling tired. You felt fit and fine. If you have gone through this phase and can remember such times, congratulations. That means that you were eating a healthy diet supported with plenty of exercise. And then your lifestyle changed. Instead of walking you decided to take the car. Instead of doing any sort of physical exercise, like swimming or jogging, you decided to spend the hours sitting crunched up in front of the computer or in front of the TV. Within six months or so, you found your posture spoiled and a distinctively visible bulging waistline. What happened to that slim, trim silhouette? Well, you really did not have the time to bother about weight loss, because you are so busy working on your job, and your first priority was to earn your living. As your bank balance increased your physical state of good health deteriorated. Until one day you found out that your legs could not carry your body up two flights of stairs without you huffing and puffing. Now how did that happen?

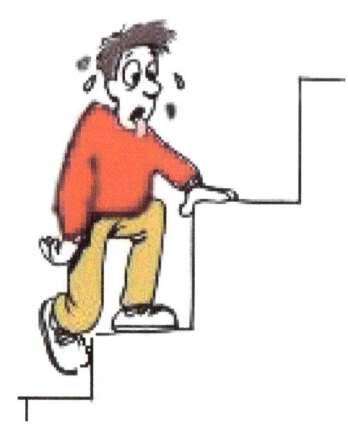

**Don't tell me there are 8 more steps still to go…**

Sunrise, sunset, sunrise, sunset, swiftly fly the years... And those years brought about a change in your physical shape. That extra layer of fat and cellulite in your 30s and 40s, when it was not present in your 10s and 20s, when you were physically active is going to affect your heart, liver, kidney and other organs. Losing weight can reduce the pressure put on these organs. Your heart will not have to work so hard, trying to pump blood through arteries, which are choked with fat cells. This is the reason why you need to lose weight.

But I hate dieting, you say. You also add that you bought this book because you wanted tips and techniques on how to lose weight without really dieting. Why have I been talking all this time without getting to what you really want to know?

Well, all this time, I was telling you about how dieting can harm you, why you need to lose weight, if you have bad eating habits inculcated during childhood and also another point – if you are genetically prone to obesity, and you have ancestors who were fat, you cannot be thin and have a pencil thin silhouette. Many people do not understand this and starve them to anorexic levels. So, if all your family members are fat and you starve yourself hoping to become slim, you are harming yourself. Eat sensibly and you will lose weight. But you are not going to be as pencil thin as some stick insect you admire. He or she has a different genetic makeup.

People suffering from hypothyroidism also find it very difficult to lose weight.

# SO NOW WE COME TO HOW TO LOSE WEIGHT WITHOUT REALLY DIETING

Do you ever find yourself in this situation?

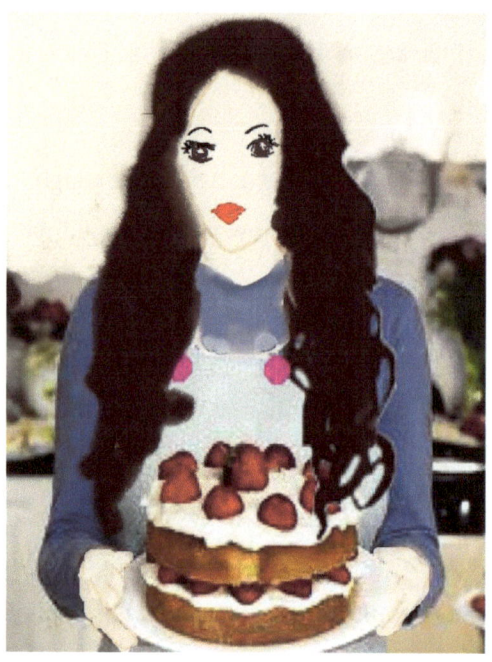

**If you love to cook, what fun is it if you cannot eat those goodies?**

If you are like a majority of us out there, the very thought of going on a diet is going to make you curl up inside. Immediate visions of boring, tasteless and monotonous diet regimes rise before your eyes. You know full well that you do really need to lose weight, but the memory of all your previous failures, all those weeks of calorie counting, portion weighing misery just makes your heart sink into your boots!

Now you are going to learn the sane approach to losing weight. I am not going to punish you by asking you to practice miracles of self-denial. In fact, I am going to encourage you to eat whatever you want, once a week – within reasonable limits; no binges please-so that you do not think that you are depriving yourself of the good things of life, namely what you deem del.icio.us food! So now, even the most fainthearted can win the battle of the bulge!

*That is because -*

Your dieting goal is – find a successful slimming method which meets with all these objects –

- Weight must be lost.

- Weight loss must not be regained again.

- The period of losing weight must not be accompanied by distressing symptoms like hunger, irritability or fatigue.

- The food you eat must consist of all the essential nutrients needed to keep your body fit and healthy.

- Losing weight must not become an obsessive and antisocial process.

- Losing weight must be simple. It should not have a taxing effect on your physical and mental well-being.

  This is what you wanted, did not you. Many people are going to say that this is well-nigh impossible. But surely we can try and get 100% successful result.

Well then, here goes –

Here is how we lose weight successfully. This is based on two important principles. Learn these principles thoroughly.

## Re-educate your eating habits

Losing weight is a question of reeducating your entire eating habits. This is not nearly so drastic as it sounds and you are going to understand that as you read on!

## The second principle is – losing weight is done slowly and has to be done slowly

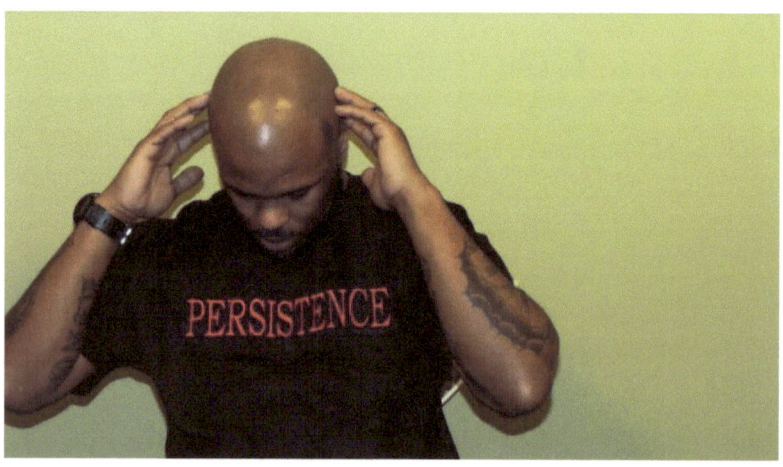

**(Photo courtesy- Mark Chase.) Mark may know that persistence pays off but how many of us have the patience to persist? But it pays to persist in the long run.**

Losing weight slowly is something that just cannot be emphasized too strongly. Weight must be lost slowly. Weight that is lost quickly is weight that is almost always put back on again. *Weight that is lost slowly is weight that is usually lost permanently.*

But what do we mean by slowly? There is no single answer to that question. What may be slow for one person may be fast for another. It may also depend on your genetic makeup. It may also depend on your age group. If you are in your 40s and 50s, and expect to be as slim and trim as you were in your 20s that is not possible. You will lose weight, but you are not going to look like a 25-year-old, unless your body has gone through plenty of restorative surgery. Remember that your physique is going to change as your body ages. So your job is to look at your age group, and implemented the tips given here accordingly. Use your common sense to know what is right for you.

Coming back to fast and slow weight loss. In general, what is meant is a loss of a mere one or 2 pounds a week, certainly not more. That means your body is getting used to this weight loss and is adjusting itself to the newer slim, trim, you. In some cases weight loss should be even less perhaps only half a pound a week. Get your doctor to look at you and advise you on how much weight you need to lose every week to hit a steady permanent constant, which he considers healthy for your state of health and age group. Then just maintain that weight.

Many of us are going to be disappointed here. We may think that we will never ever get down to our desirable weight, if we have to lose anywhere between half a pound – two pounds every week. But this is easier than you think.

Look at this example –

Supposing you are 28 pounds overweight. 14 weeks is all it takes to remove all that excessive avoirdupois. This is just over three months. A weight loss of 1 pound a week in six months and that is very little time. Indeed, especially when you consider all the time it takes to lose weight with strict conventional diets, when you then lose heart, pile all the weight back on again, and then start all over again.

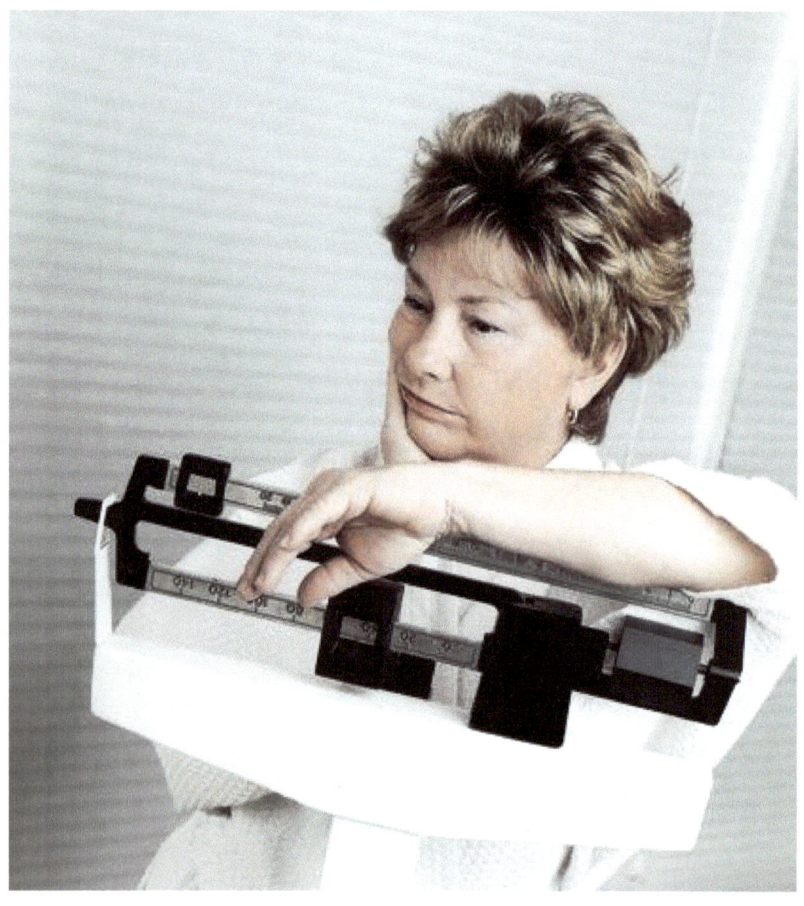

**Is that you? If you find yourself stepping on the weighing machine every 12 hours, stop please!**

Many people spend years, maybe even a lifetime trying to lose weight unsuccessfully. But here you are, losing 28 pounds in three months? Is not that wonderful?

Also don't think that you'll lose weight overnight or within the next 48 hours. If that happens suddenly, there is something wrong in your system somewhere…

These two principles that you have just learned are not entirely separate. In fact, they have a common link. This is the link which is the actual method by which you lose weight.

So now we come to brass tacks.

To lose weight, all you need to do is to eat a little less. Just a little less, please, not a lot less. Two potatoes instead of three. Hey, I am talking about potatoes. You are supposed to be losing weight. Are not potatoes, a no-no for those people intending to lose weight, you say.

I told you, I am not going to tell you not to eat the food you like. I am making this a fun session. I am giving you tips to keep you healthy. You like potatoes. I like potatoes. Everyone likes potatoes. But thanks to some strict joyless dietitians, we have cut them out of our daily diets, thus depriving ourselves of delicious boiled and baked potatoes with garlic salt and herbs dribbled all over them. We are not going to do that. So we are going to eat them to our hearts content. But we are not going to eat four potatoes as we did yesterday. We are going to eat three potatoes. Maybe six months from now, we are going to eat 2 ½ potatoes. That depends on how hungry we feel. We are definitely not going to deprive our bodies of the things we like best. In the same way, we are going to eat one slice of toast instead of two. With two exceptions [I am going to describe them in a moment,] **do not change the food you eat or the drinks you drink.**

Shocked? This is a revolutionary idea. But well then, my intention is to keep you healthy and to keep you happy. So never mind if people tell you that that piece of cake or that bar of chocolate is full of calories.

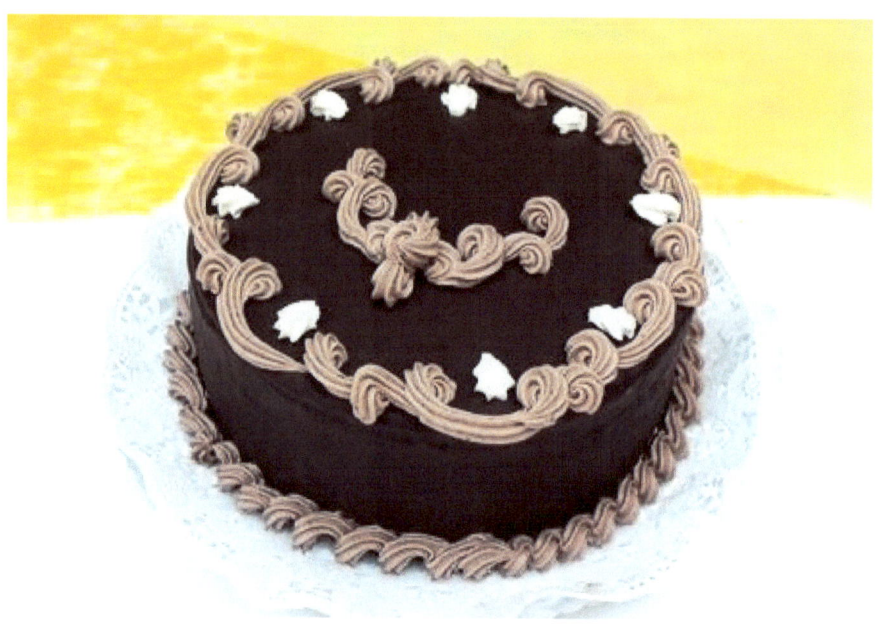

**If you like the cake or the chocolate then eat it. But only have a little less of chocolate or cake or éclairs than what you had previously.**

**HERE ARE THE TWO EXCEPTIONS –**

The two exceptions to the basic principles that you do not need to change your food are these –

Reduce your fried food intake. If you like fried bacon or fried eggs, try poaching them and grilling them instead. You may even want to bake the eggs. You are saving 80 – hundred calories per portion and your food is as delicious as it was before. If you really need to fry something, fry the food in a nonstick pan, in the food's own fat. That means you are not adding extra fat to that which is already present in the food. There was a time when you pre-fried vegetables in fat when you made minced meat dishes. Well, fry the meat in its own fat and then add the vegetables in this cooked mixture. Simmer slowly and enjoy.

The second exception is known to everybody who is bothered about weight loss. No sugar. Try sweetening your pancakes with no calorie sweetening powder if you have a sweet tooth. Anything which has corn syrup in it should be avoided like the plague.

Now, here I come to a point which is going to make all the soft drink companies hungry for my hemoglobin. Stop drinking artificial sweetened cold drinks like Coca-Cola and Pepsi. Let me tell you the story of how a popular singer of yesteryear, Rod Stewart found out all about the power of Coca-Cola. Coca-Cola originated as a digestive drink. You needed to take just two spoons to help you digest your food. But here are we, chugging bottles of Coca-Cola at one time. Now, Rod Stewart was an employee of Coca-Cola, before "blondes have more fun" made history. During an interview, he said he had to inspect a Coca-Cola Vat. He leaned over it, and his ball pen slipped and fell inside it. Six months later the vat was cleaned. *The plastic covering of the ball pen had been totally eaten away. Only the metal portion was left.*, so just imagine what these drinks are doing to your innards, especially when you give them to your children ever so often. Try fresh fruit juice instead, not concentrated juice. That is always the healthiest option.

You will probably agree that these two exceptions do not materially change the food and drink that you consume, but you do not know how your body is going to bless you for this food change.

All those tiny little bits of food that you are not eating add up to weight. So you not eating that food means no extra weight gain. Logical, is not it?

Only a small amount of weight is going to be "not put on", but over a period of a few weeks, you are going to see a visible weight loss. At the same time as you have been losing weight slowly, you have been reeducating your eating habits. You will soon find that you do not crave sugar because your body has got used to doing without it, and has changed your biochemical and biophysical logical system accordingly.

However, your body needs a little bit of sugar in order to keep functioning properly. Try Honey. Also try eating more fruit. Fruit sugar is natural sugar. Your body is going to assimilate it better.

Now you happen to be suffering from a sweet tooth. How does an eating of smaller portions of two chocolate biscuits – 170 cal – help you lose weight? You eat one biscuit. You save 85 cal. Sweet tasting foods are eaten almost entirely for their taste, so just bite off a little piece of chocolate or cake and chew slowly, savoring the flavor and taste. Then eat another tiny piece of chocolate. Believe it or not, by the time you eat half a bar of chocolate, you will feel as if you have had enough. That is because the flavor has been in your mouth for a longer while. It is also equal to two or three whole chocolates gulped down in large mouthfuls. Try it out right now.

I am stressing one point again here – it is absolutely not necessary for you to count calories when you are eating your food, and thus take all the fun out of enjoying your meals. How many times have you heard your friends mourn "I would love to have that, but it has so many calories?" Just walk up to them. Ask them the portions size they would like to eat, if they were not bothered about calories.

"One slice of chocolate pastry, how delicious it looks, " they are going to say. Pick up the chocolate pastry. Cut it into two. Remove one portion. [You may finish it off yourself.] Ask them to eat the half, even though they keep protesting about calories. Tell them to eat small bites. They are going to bless you for taking the decision of "to eat or not to eat – that is the question." out of their hands. Tell them that you know of what you do. Tell them they do not need to feel guilty. Tell them to enjoy that chocolate pastry. Do not blame me if you find your friend circle expanding monumentally and you are voted the best friend a guy/girl could ever have!

There is plenty of applied psychology in weight loss. These tips and techniques given are based on common sense and applied psychology!

**Find motivation to lose weight!**

**If you are motivated enough, half the battle is won!**

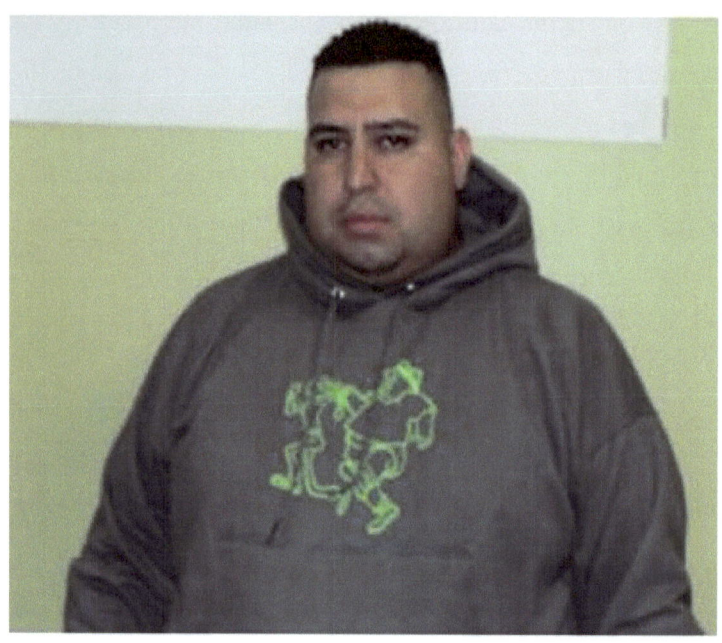

**(Photo Courtesy: Joel)  Joel has the Will power and motivation to lose weight. I know he'll do it. After all his sweatshirt says it all!**

# Easy Tips and Techniques to Remain Slim and Trim

## Let us help you get started with easy tips and techniques to remain Slim and trim.

Always eat your food when you are seated at a table. Never allow any solid food to pass through your lips that cannot be eaten using a knife, fork or spoon. This psychological ploy is to ensure that you never eat food without actively thinking about it. It is surprising how often many of us will eat almost anything as the subconscious act or just for something to do. Never eat food, when you are bored or when your attention is diverted elsewhere, for example, watching television. I am giving just one exception here – food eaten while watching a sport outdoors. As long as the sandwiches are full of cheese, green leafy vegetables, one slice of cooked ham or grilled bacon, tomatoes, sprinkled with herbs and made up of whole wheat or multigrain breads, you have one food item from all the food pyramids here. Grill the sandwiches to cook them or make hamburgers out of them. So enjoy the baseball game and enjoy your food too!

Do not be afraid to refuse an extra portion. It is not bad manners to refuse food, especially when the hostess is intent on piling up your plate. But there are exceptions to the rule here – if you are in the East, and you refuse food offered to you, the hostess is going to feel hurt. She is going to think that her dinner is not good enough, because you are not eating lots and lots of food. So at the first instance, take a small helping of maybe say 2 teaspoons. When she says take more, take another small helping of another teaspoon. Honor is satisfied on both counts!

I asked a French friend of mine how he managed to keep his weight within control, especially when he had to eat and drink a lot on many social occasions. He gave me a very sensible answer – he said, "before I begin eating, I ask one of the waiters to overload a plate with everything on it and place it in front of me. I look at the plate. My mind says, "if you eat all that, you are really going to feel sick. You are also going to ruin your health." So with the plate still in front of me, I pick up another plate. I then look at the items that I find most appetizing. I then take small portions of those items. Just enough for a taste. If they are good, I take another small portion. After I have finished one round, I taste the second round of the items I left out in the first round. The portions are even smaller. Well, I have eaten a full meal, and I have eaten well. I have enjoyed my food. I have enjoyed the party. Is that not good."

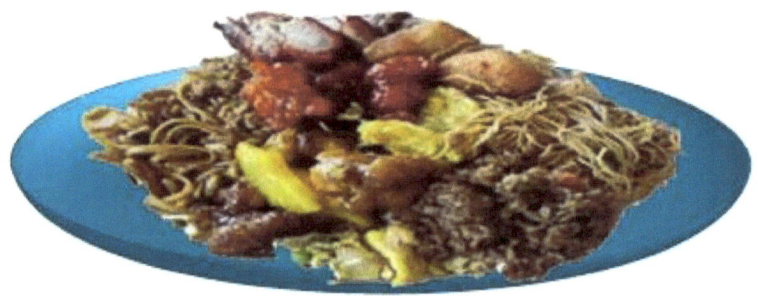

**There is no reason why you should not enjoy what you like as long as your health (and your doctor) permits. But a less overflowing plate- Smaller portions!- please.**

I thought that this was the most sensible advice given to me by a most sensible person. He is 70 years old now. He is fit, he is fine. He is known as a gourmet and connoisseur of good food and drink. And best of all, he does not stint on the foods he loves. Don't you think that this is a good way to live life Emperor Size?

Also, he told me one thing. Eat off a smaller plate. The visual perception of food has a lot to do with satisfying hunger. That is why he asks waiters to overload a plate beforehand! A small plate of food, which can be just as stimulating to the hungry appetite as a large plateful, will often satisfy hunger equally well.

Have you seen Barbra Streisand in the Mirror Has Two Faces? Jeff Bridges watches her eat the perfect mouthful. She cuts her food up in small pieces. And then she makes different combinations of different ingredients. All of these combinations are perfect for her. Well, she has found out the best idea of how to remain Slim and trim while enjoying everything she loves to eat! Also, the plateful of small pieces makes it look as if there are lots and lots of food on your plate. Also, you are going to pick up all those pieces and enjoy them. You will be surprised how much this helps you to savor the full flavor of food, even though they are smaller portions.

Limit the time you allow yourself to eat your meal. You need to have four meals a day without fail. No compromise here. I have seen a number of people stinting on their meals under the impression that if they miss a meal, they are going to lose weight. Definitely not advised. Not only are you not going to lose weight, but you are going to put on weight. That is because you have starved your body. It is in desperation mode. The mind says "there is no food source easily available, because meals are being missed. So start storing fat on which the body can subsist if it starts to starve. "Believe me, this is true, and this is a natural phenomenon. Also, if your body is not kept well hydrated with plenty of fresh juice or water throughout the day, the body is again going to go into "store water instead of elimination" mode. That is all the extra weight, which is lost temporarily if you go in for some detoxification diet without healthy nutrients, proteins and carbohydrates. But then the body is in panic mode. It puts on weight so that it can survive.

Do not gulp down your food in a hurry. How come the aristocrats of yore had 20 course banquets, but still managed to keep fit and fine? That is because they took their time in eating. They took small portions. They ate those portions slowly. And then they gave their bodies time to digest the food, before they started on round two of eating and drinking. They also exercised regularly. They were good warriors, hunters and riders. They never sat down in places for more than 10 minutes. They were always up and about. That is why their body systems allowed them to assimilate food really quickly, to get ready for the next round.

Well, we do not sit down regularly to 4-5 courses meals. That would finish us off, thanks to our sedentary lifestyles and lack of exercise. Nevertheless, with just a little bit of lifestyle change right now, we can find ourselves losing weight really successfully and easily.

Also, if they drank, they drank in moderation. Drinks were just used to keep the body dehydrated and not as something which he used as an artificial support, just because your life was insupportable. They really did not have time to bother about self-analysis. The thinking modern man has become so introspective, that he spends more time wondering why he feels some way, why he should feel that way, what made him feel that way or anything else which allows him to discuss his problems with everybody around him. There was a time when people did not bother much about such self-indulgent introspectiveness. They just went out if they were feeling blue and indulged in healthy physical exercise. That banished all the gloomy feelings.

But the modern man would rather lie down on the psychologists couch and talk and talk and talk. In fact, parents are also asking psychological opinions of their children and asking for advice. This is a very dangerous trend. It needs to be stopped. Healthy living means a healthy body. It also means a healthy mind. A healthy mind can only be cultivated through good diet, less of psychology, a disciplined lifestyle and sensible, intelligent and experienced adults and advisors around you when you were a child!

# Conclusion

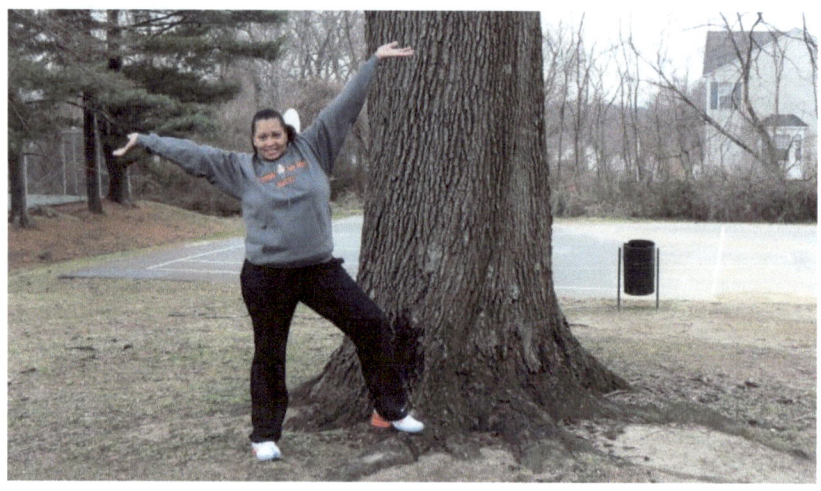

**Life is Good! Natasha is Getting her Sexy back!**

These are just some of the tips and techniques which have been passed down through ancient times, in order to keep you healthy, fit and fine. All of them can be implemented in your lifestyle without you going through life altering changes! Here I want to emphasize that most of you will not need them eating of fraction less in each meal soon become second nature, and the result is that very soon you will be eating all the foods that you enjoy eating. You will not be counting calories. You will be eating healthily. You will be eating and drinking happily. And you will be losing weight without *really* dieting!

# Author Bio

**Dueep Jyot Singh** is a Management and IT Professional who managed to gather Postgraduate qualifications in Management and English and Degrees in Science, French and Education while pursuing different enjoyable career options like being an hospital administrator, IT,SEO and HRD Database Manager/ trainer, movie scriptwriter, theatre artiste and public speaker, lecturer in French, Marketing and Advertising, ex-Editor of Hearts On Fire (now known as Solctice) Books Missouri USA, advice columnist and cartoonist, publisher and Aviation School trainer, ex- moderator on Medico.in, banker, student councilor ,travelogue writer … among other things! One fine morning, she decided that she had enough of killing herself by Degrees and went back to her first love -- writing. It's more enjoyable! She already has 24 published academic and 11 fiction- in- different- genre books under her belt.

When she is not designing websites or making Graphic design illustrations for clients who want Walt Disney, Norman Rockwell , JJ Grandville or Hed Kandy type illustrations, she is busy browsing in old bookshops for antique books,-she has a mouthwatering collection of priceless First editions and rare books…including R.L. Stevenson, O.Henry, Dornford Yates, Maurice Walsh, C.N.Williamson, and the crown of her collection- Dickens "The Old Curiosity Shop," and so on… Just call her "Renaissance Woman" - collecting herbal remedies, making one of a kind creations in Irish Crochet and Aran knitting, acting like Universal Helping Hand/Agony Aunt, or escaping to her dear mountains for a bit of exploring, collecting herbs and plants , trekking, and rappelling.

Check out some of the other JD-Biz Publishing books

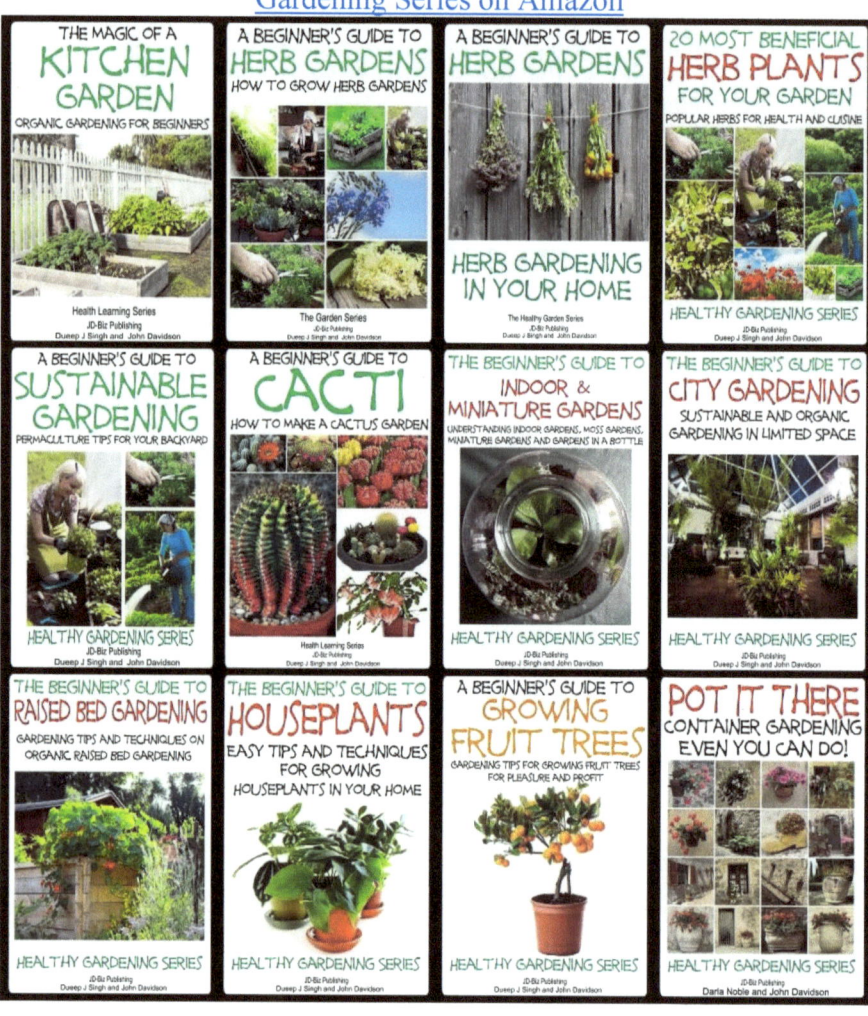

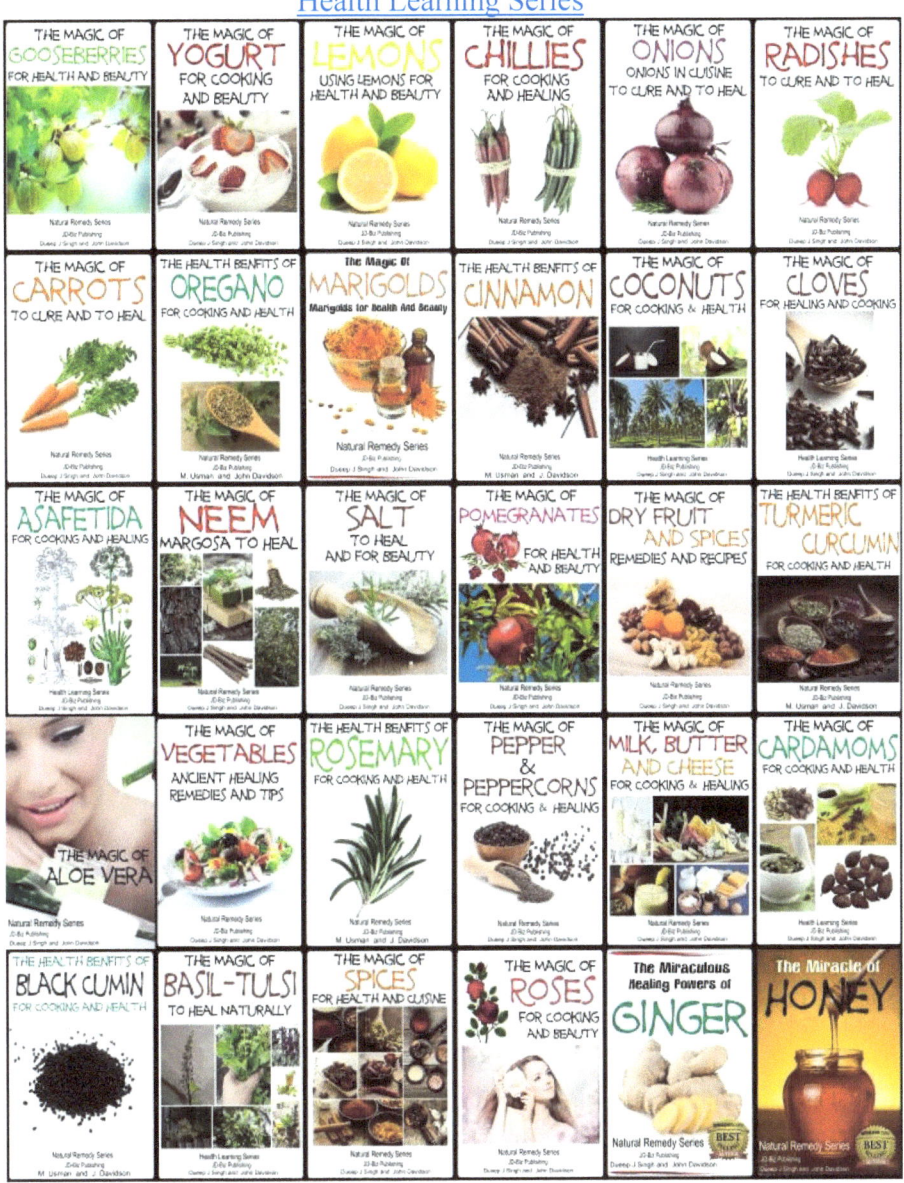

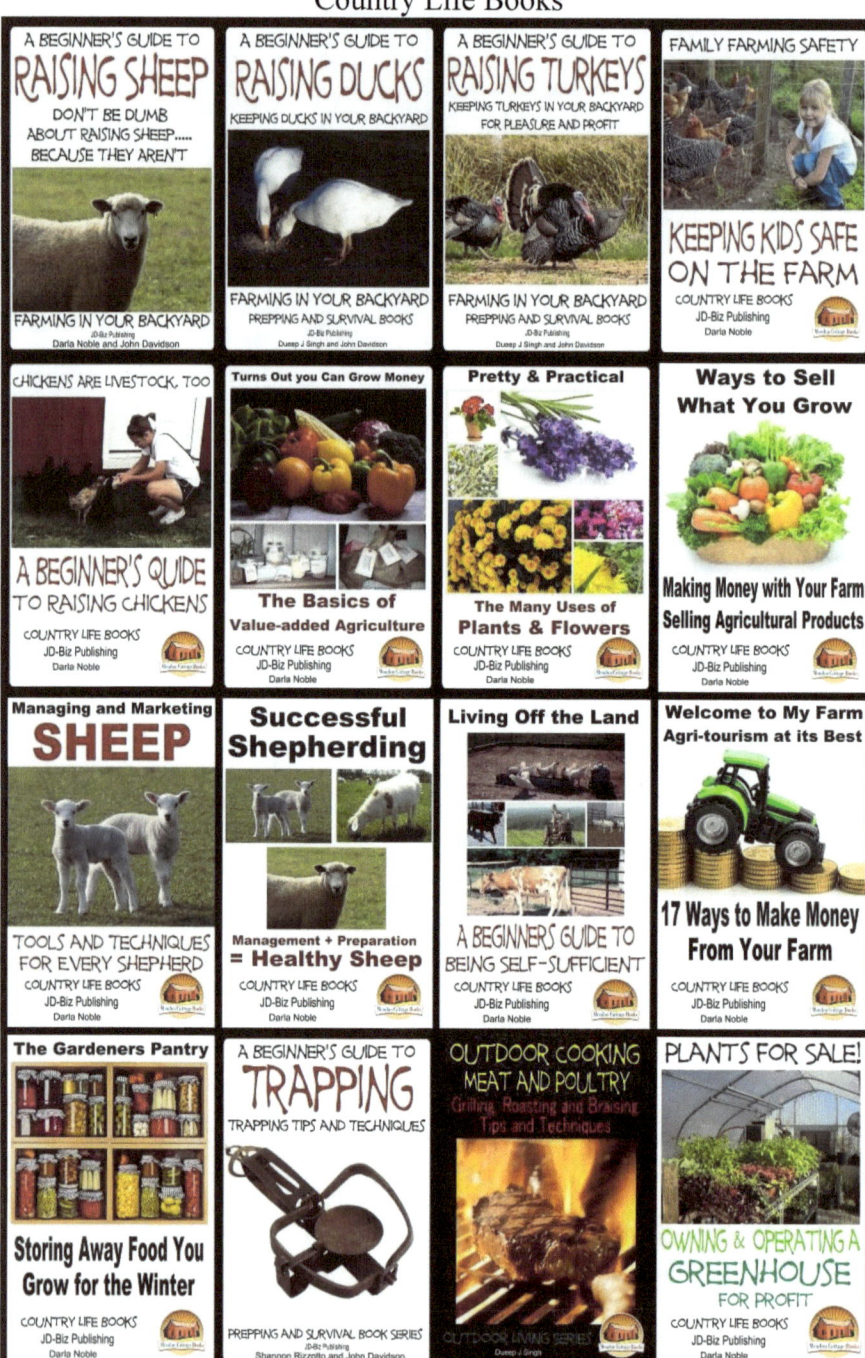

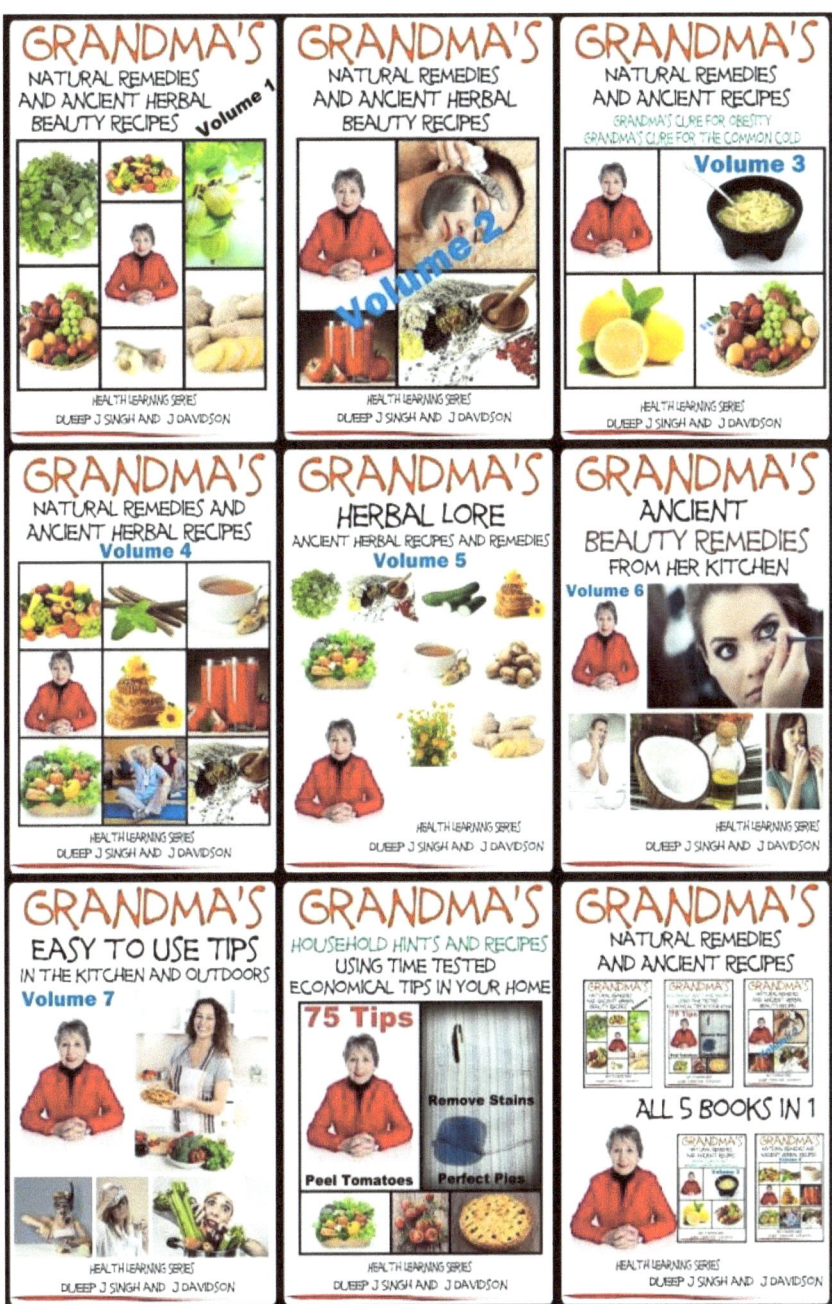

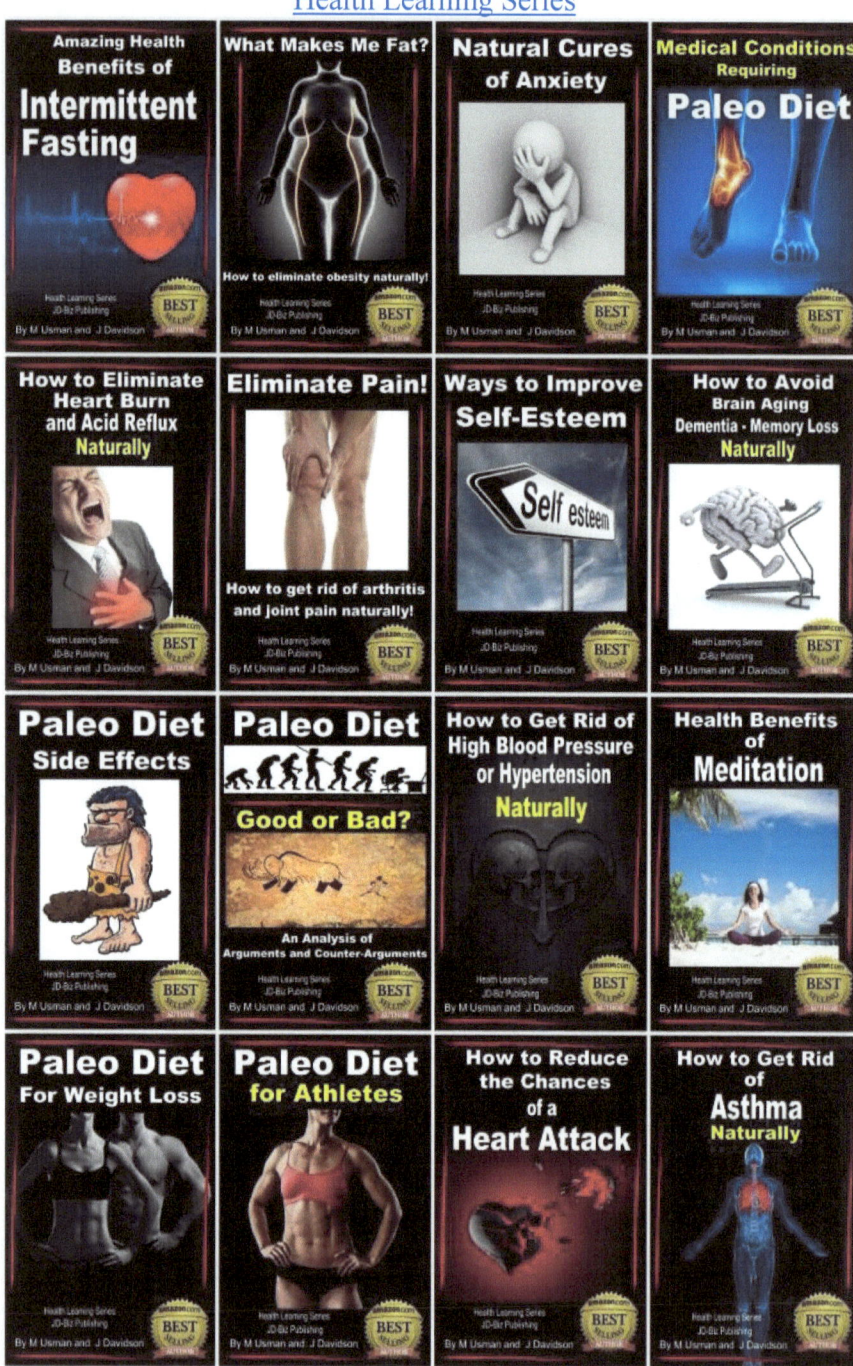

Amazing Animal Book Series

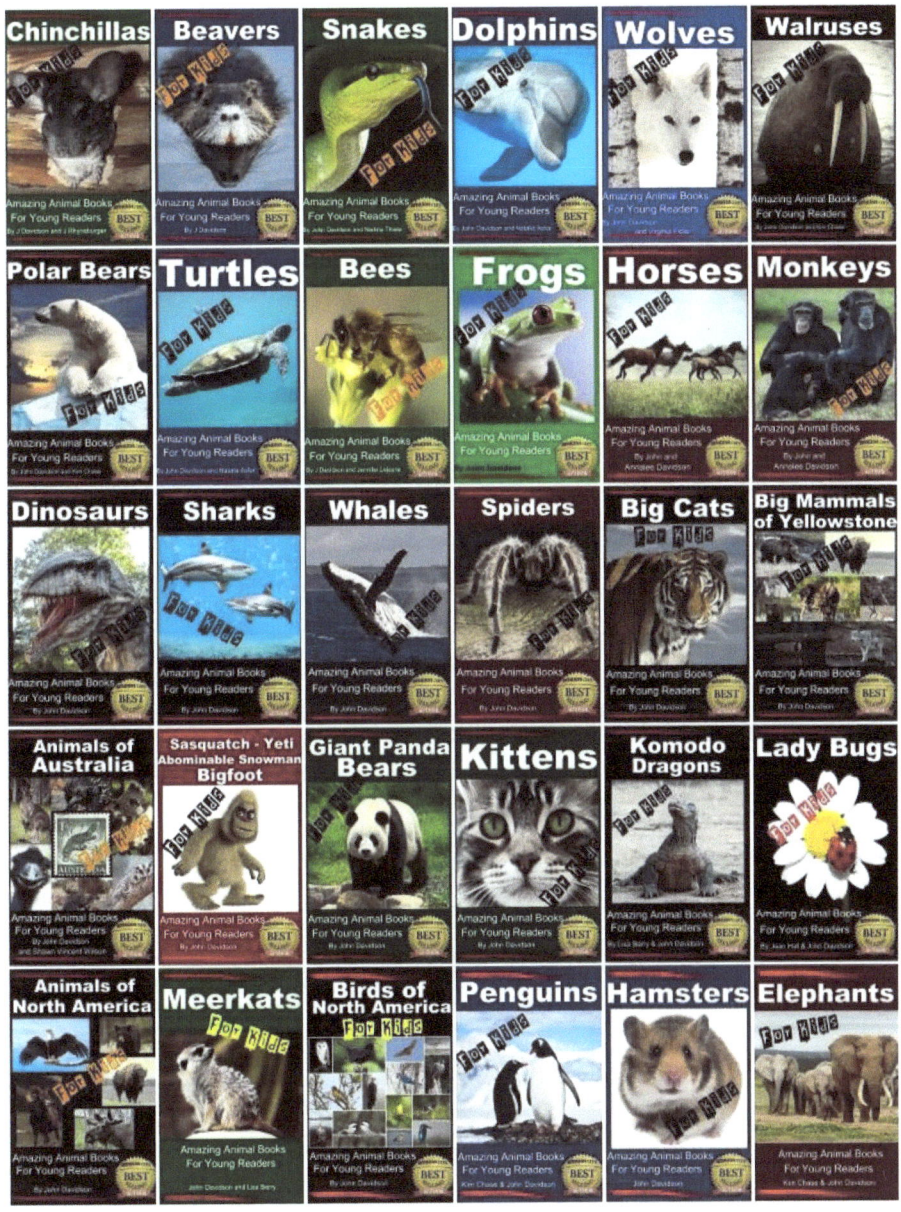

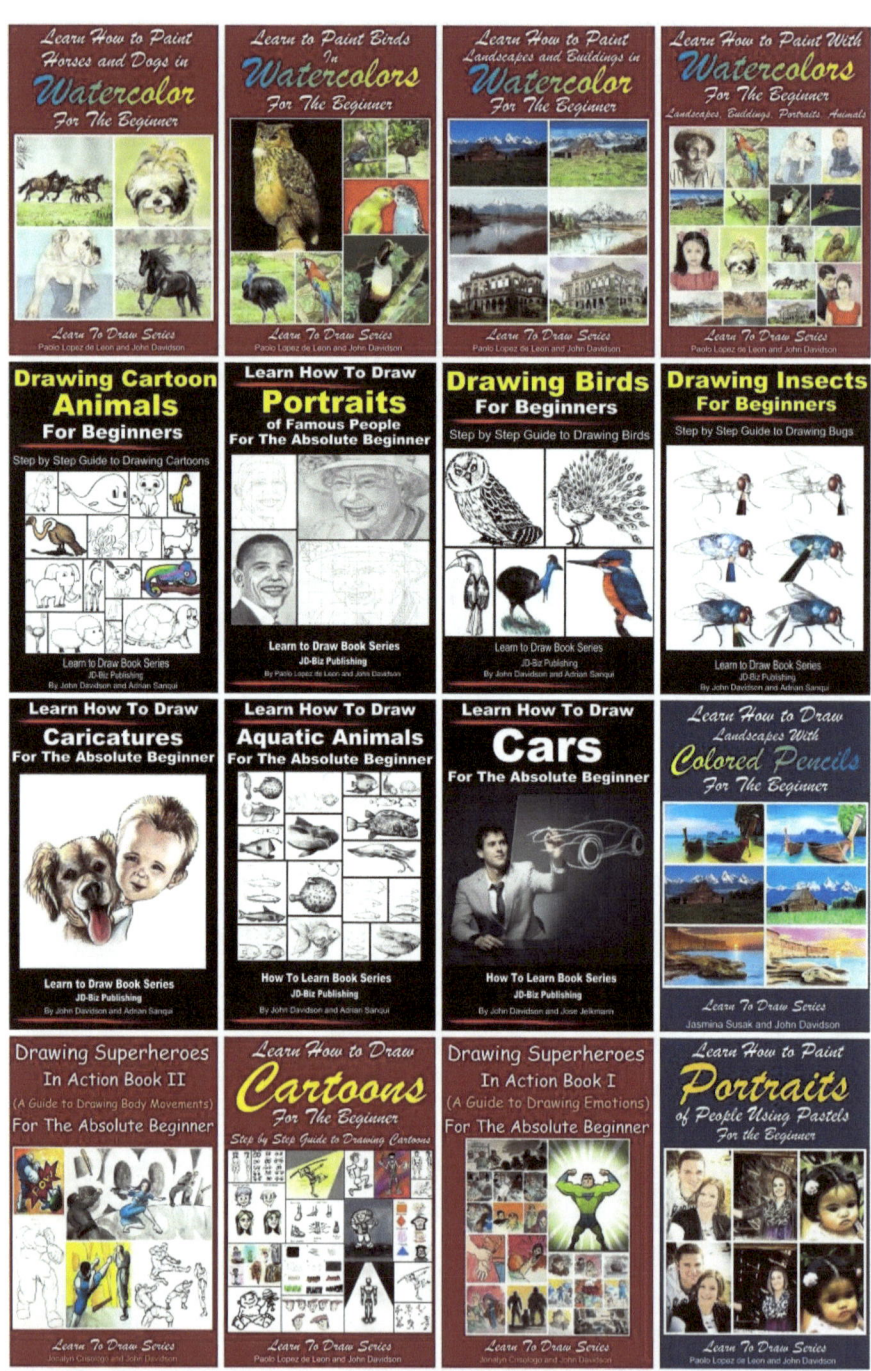

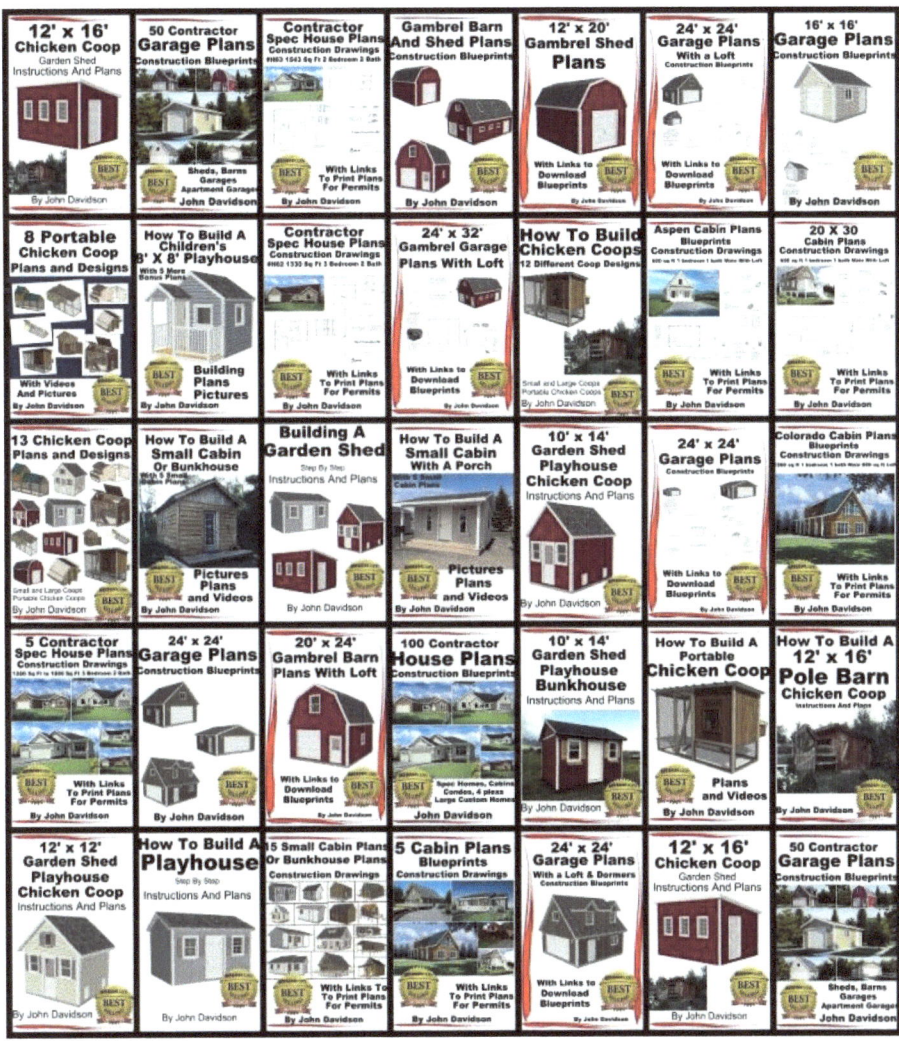

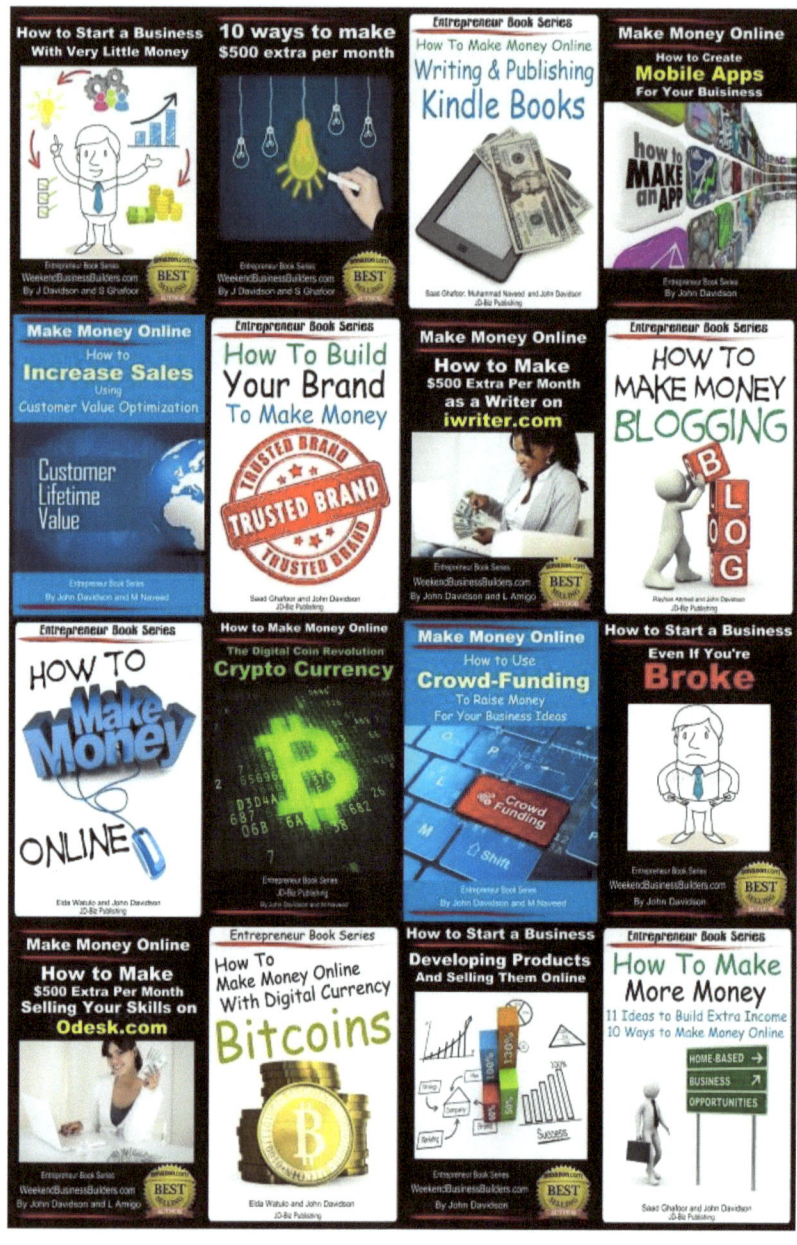

**Our books are available at**

1. Amazon.com
2. Barnes and Noble
3. Itunes
4. Kobo
5. Smashwords
6. Google Play Books


## Download Free Books!

## http://MendonCottageBooks.com

# Publisher

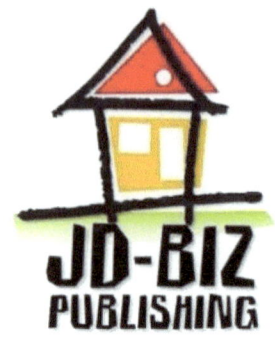

JD-Biz Corp

P O Box 374

Mendon, Utah 84325

http://www.jd-biz.com/

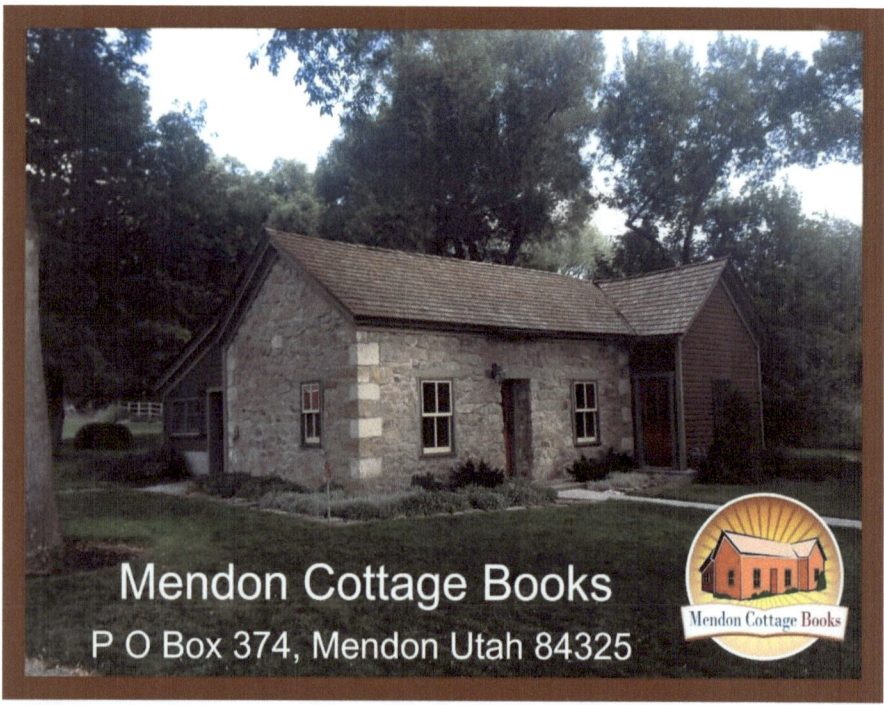

www.ingramcontent.com/pod-product-compliance
Lightning Source LLC
Chambersburg PA
CBHW050841290526
45792CB00001B/480